Stretching Exercises for Seniors

36 Effective Workouts to Stay Fit and Build Core Strength

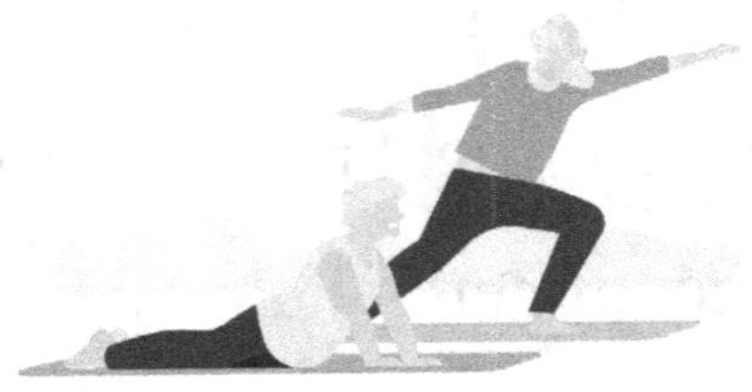

Everly Brooks

Table of Contents

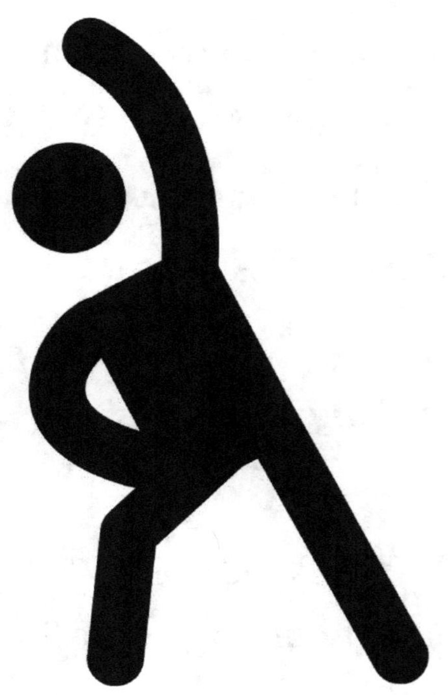

Introduction

As the morning sun gently peeked through the curtains, casting a warm glow across the room, a sense of awakening filled the air. The topic of conversation today is **stretching exercises for seniors**—a powerful tool to embrace a vibrant and active life, regardless of age.

Why Stretching Exercises are Important for Seniors:

In the ever-changing tapestry of life, our bodies naturally undergo transformations as we age. Muscles may lose some of their flexibility, and joints can become less supple. However, within these changes lies an invitation—an opportunity to rediscover the strength that resides within and to nurture a healthier, more vibrant self.

Stretching exercises hold a special place in the hearts of seniors. They are not merely about touching your toes or reaching for the sky; instead, they are a profound act of self-love. It's a way to honor your body's journey, acknowledging the miles it has carried you and the stories it holds within.

Benefits of Stretching for Overall Health and Core Strength:

Now, let's explore the remarkable benefits that await you on this stretching journey. Picture this: with each gentle stretch, you open the door to a world of possibilities -possibilities of better health, increased mobility, and enhanced core strength.

Stretching exercises can alleviate those nagging aches and pains, providing comfort to your body as it gracefully adapts to the challenges of aging. They enhance blood circulation, nurturing your muscles with the oxygen they crave and bringing a renewed sense of energy.

Beyond the physical aspects, stretching exercises open a gateway to emotional and mental well-being. As you embark on this journey, you'll find moments of tranquility and mindfulness, where stress dissipates like morning mist, leaving you with a calm, centered mind.

This book, ***"Stretching Exercises for Seniors,"*** is more than just a collection of exercises. It's a heartfelt invitation to embrace the beauty of life, to listen to the symphony of your body, and to step into a world of strength, vitality, and joy.

Within the following chapters, you will discover 35 effective workouts specially designed for seniors like you. These exercises will be your companions as you explore newfound realms of possibility, nurturing your body, mind, and soul.

Before you embark on this journey, take a moment to acknowledge your own unique story, for within it lies the courage to begin anew. With each page you turn, may you find inspiration, wisdom, and empowerment to stay fit, improve your health, and build the core strength that will carry you through life's every twist and turn.

Welcome to "Stretching Exercises for Seniors"—where the power of stretching meets the beauty of the human spirit. Let's embark on this empowering adventure together!

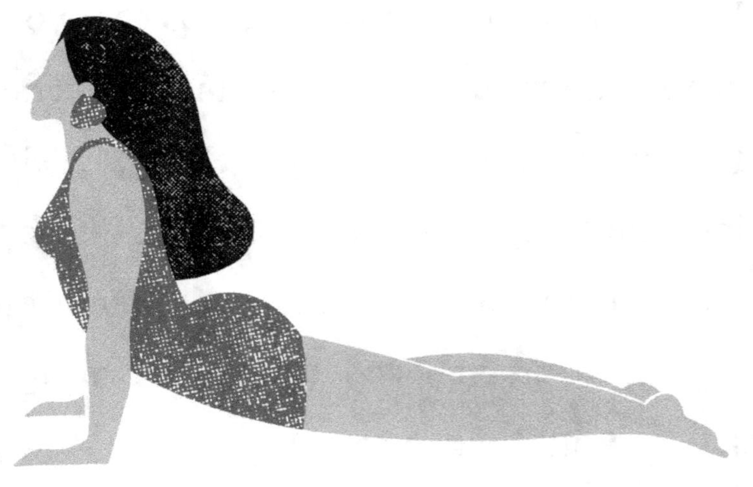

Getting Started

In the early hours of the day, as the world begins to stir, it's time to lay the foundation for your stretching journey. Before we delve into the invigorating stretches, let's take a moment to prepare and understand our bodies—a crucial step towards ensuring a safe and fulfilling experience.

Preparing for Stretching Exercises:

Like an artist preparing their canvas, getting ready for stretching exercises sets the stage for an enriching experience. Here are some essential steps to consider before you begin:

1. **Create a Calm Space:** Find a quiet and comfortable space where you can focus without distractions. A serene environment enhances your mind-body connection during stretches.

2. **Warm-Up Routines:** Before diving into deep stretches, warm up your body with gentle movements. These preliminary exercises increase blood flow to your muscles, making them more receptive to stretching.

3. **Dress Comfortably:** Wear loose, breathable clothing that allows for unrestricted movement. This ensures you

can fully engage in each stretch without feeling constricted.

4. **Gather Necessary Equipment:** In most cases, stretching exercises require no equipment. However, having a yoga mat or a soft surface can provide added comfort during floor-based stretches.

5. **Stay Hydrated:** Hydration is essential for overall health and flexibility. Make sure to drink enough water before and after your stretching sessions.

Just as each person has a unique fingerprint, our bodies possess individual needs and limitations. Understanding and respecting these aspects are paramount to a safe and effective stretching routine:

1. **Listen to Your Body:** Your body communicates with you in subtle ways. Pay attention to how it feels during each stretch. If you experience pain or discomfort, adjust the intensity or modify the movement accordingly.

2. **Know Your Range of Motion:** We all have different levels of flexibility. Embrace

your current range of motion without comparing it to others. Gradually, with consistent practice, you may notice improvements.

3. **Respect Your Joints:** Be mindful of your joints' limitations, especially if you have any pre-existing conditions like arthritis. Avoid overstretching or putting excessive pressure on vulnerable areas.

4. **Consult a Professional:** If you have specific health concerns or medical conditions, consider consulting a healthcare provider or a fitness expert before beginning any new exercise program.

5. **Be Patient and Gentle:** Rome wasn't built in a day, and neither will your flexibility. Be patient with yourself and embrace progress at your own pace. Gentle, gradual stretches yield long-lasting results.

Remember, the journey of stretching exercises is not a race to achieve perfection but a dance of self-discovery. As you prepare and understand your body's unique needs, you cultivate a deeper connection with yourself, embracing the beauty of self-care and growth.

Now that we have laid the groundwork, let's venture into the heart of our stretching adventure. The upcoming chapters will unveil a plethora of exercises designed to invigorate your body, mind, and soul. So, take a deep breath, and let the journey begin!

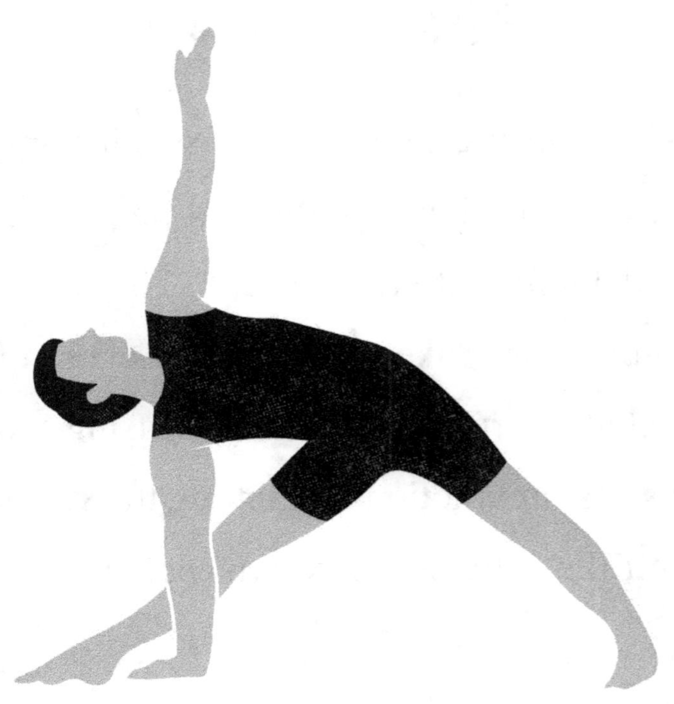

Warm-Up Routines

As the sun rises higher in the sky, it's time to awaken your body gently and prepare it for the delightful stretches ahead. The warm-up routines are like the first strokes of a painter's brush, gradually easing your muscles into motion and setting the stage for a fulfilling stretching experience.

GENTLE WARM-UP EXERCISES TO LOOSEN MUSCLES:

1. **Neck Rolls:** Begin by sitting or standing with your shoulders relaxed. Slowly roll your head to one side, bringing your ear towards your shoulder. Hold for a few

seconds, feeling the stretch along the side of your neck. Repeat on the other side.

2. **Shoulder Circles:** Stand tall with your feet shoulder-width apart. Roll your shoulders forward in big circles, then switch to backward circles. These movements help loosen up the shoulder joints and release tension.

3. **Arm Swings:** Extend your arms out to the sides. Swing them gently forward and backward, like you're reaching for something in front and behind you. Feel the stretch across your chest and upper back.

4. **Spine Twist:** Sit or stand with your back straight. Gently twist your upper body to one side, using your core muscles to support the movement. Hold for a moment, then twist to the other side.

PREPARING YOUR BODY FOR MORE INTENSE STRETCHING:

1. **Cat-Cow Stretch:** Begin on your hands and knees in a tabletop position. Arch your back upwards like a cat, tucking your chin to your chest. Then, drop your belly towards the floor, lifting your head and tailbone like a cow. Flow between these two positions to warm up your spine.

2. **Hip Circles:** Stand with your feet hip-width apart. Place your hands on your hips and make slow circles with your hips in one direction, then switch to the other direction. This movement helps loosen your hip joints.

3. **Leg Swings:** Hold onto a sturdy surface for support. Swing one leg gently forward and backward like a pendulum. Repeat on the other leg. This warms up your leg muscles and improves hip flexibility.

4. **Ankle Circles:** Sit or stand with your feet flat on the ground. Lift one foot slightly off the floor and rotate your ankle in circles. Repeat in the opposite direction, then switch

to the other foot. This warms up your ankles and feet.

As you perform these gentle warm-up exercises, be present in the moment, and listen to your body's cues. Allow your breath to flow naturally, syncing it with each movement. The warm-up routines serve not only to loosen your muscles but also to prepare your mind for the stretching journey ahead.

By engaging in these preparatory movements, you provide your body with the necessary care and attention it deserves. A well-warmed body is more receptive to stretching, reducing the risk of injury and enhancing the overall effectiveness of your stretching routine.

Now that you've laid the groundwork with the warm-up routines, it's time to embrace the heart of stretching exercises. In the upcoming chapters, we will explore various stretches that will invigorate your body, improve flexibility, and nourish your well-being. Get ready to discover the beauty of stretching for you, one gentle movement at a time. Let's continue our empowering journey together!

Upper Body Stretches

Here, we will focus on stretches that bring rejuvenation and flexibility to your upper body. These stretches are designed to target the shoulders, neck, arms, wrists, chest, and back, helping you find relief from tension and improve overall mobility. Let's embark on this journey of ease and relaxation.

1. Shoulder and Neck Stretches:

a. Shoulder Rolls: Sit or stand with your back straight. Slowly roll your shoulders in a circular motion—up, back, down, and forward. This gentle movement releases tension in your shoulder muscles.

b. **Neck Tilts:** Sit or stand in a comfortable position. Gently tilt your head to one side, bringing your ear towards your shoulder. Hold for a few seconds, feeling the stretch along your neck. Repeat on the other side.

2. ARM AND WRIST STRETCHES:

a. **Arm Cross Stretch:** Extend one arm in front of you and bring it across your chest. Use your other hand to gently press the extended arm closer to your body. Feel the stretch along the back of your shoulder. Repeat on the other arm.

b. **Wrist Circles:** Extend your arms in front of you, palms facing down. Make slow circles with your wrists in one direction, then switch to the other direction. This stretch helps improve wrist flexibility.

3. Chest and Back Stretches:

a. **Chest Opener:** Stand tall with your feet hip-width apart. Clasp your hands behind your back and straighten your arms. Lift your arms slightly and open your chest, squeezing your shoulder blades together. Hold for a few seconds, then release.

b. **Cat-Cow Stretch (Modified):** Sit on a chair with your feet flat on the ground. Place your hands on your knees. Inhale as you arch your back, lifting your chest and chin (Cow position). Exhale as you round your back, dropping your head (Cat position). Flow between these two positions to stretch your spine gently.

Remember to breathe deeply and relax into each stretch. Avoid forcing your body into uncomfortable positions and aim for a mild to moderate stretch sensation. With regular practice, you'll notice improved flexibility and reduced stiffness in your upper body.

As you embark on these upper body stretches, always listen to your body's signals. If you experience pain or discomfort, adjust the stretches or stop if necessary. Our goal is to nurture your body and promote well-being, and these stretches are an excellent step towards achieving that.

We'll continue to explore stretches that will benefit your lower body, core strength, and overall vitality. Keep embracing this journey with curiosity and self-compassion. Your body will thank you for the care and attention you give it. Let's continue our stretching adventure together!

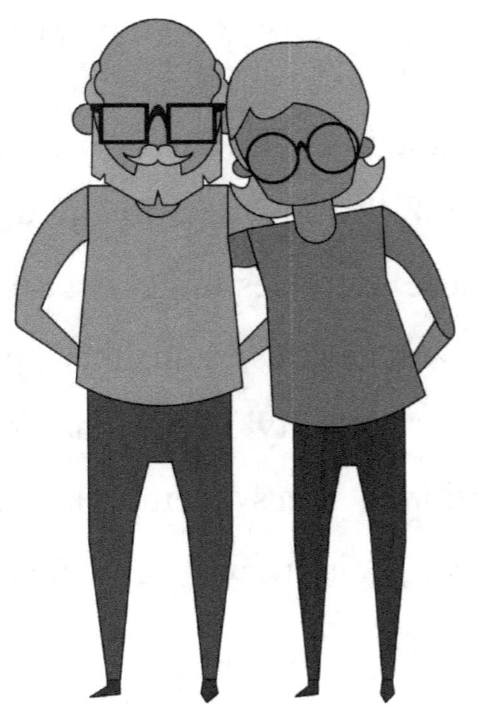

Lower Body Stretches

In this chapter, we'll delve into stretches that bring flexibility and vitality to your lower body. These exercises target the hips, thighs, legs, calves, ankles, and feet, promoting improved mobility and a sense of rejuvenation. Let's embark on this empowering journey of lower body stretches.

1. Hip and Thigh Stretches:

a. **Seated Hip Opener:** Sit on the edge of a sturdy chair with your feet flat on the floor. Cross your right ankle over your left knee, forming a figure-four shape. Gently press down on your right knee to feel the stretch in your right hip and thigh. Repeat on the other side.

b. **Standing Quadriceps Stretch:** Stand tall with your feet hip-width apart. Bend your right knee, bringing your heel towards your glutes. Hold your right ankle with your right hand, feeling the stretch in your quadriceps. Repeat on the other leg.

2. Leg and Calf Stretches:

a. **Standing Hamstring Stretch:** Stand tall with your feet hip-width apart. Extend your right leg forward and flex your foot. Hinge at your hips, reaching towards your right foot with both hands. Feel the stretch in your hamstrings. Repeat on the other leg.

b. **Calf Stretch (Wall Push):** Stand facing a wall, with your hands pressed against it. Step your right foot back and keep your heel on the floor. Bend your left knee and lean forward to feel the stretch in your right calf. Repeat on the other leg.

3. Ankle and Foot Stretches:

a. **Ankle Circles:** Sit on a chair with your feet flat on the floor. Lift one foot off the ground and make slow circles with your ankle in one direction, then switch to the other direction. This stretch enhances ankle flexibility.

b. **Toe Stretch:** Sit on a chair with your feet flat on the floor. Lift your right foot and curl your toes inward, then extend them outward. This stretch helps improve foot mobility and relieves tension.

Remember to perform these stretches gently and with awareness. Never push your body beyond its limits, and focus on maintaining steady breath throughout each stretch. With regular practice, you'll experience increased flexibility and reduced stiffness in your lower body.

As you engage in these lower body stretches, cherish the connection between your mind and body. Embrace the sensations, and use each stretch as an opportunity to cultivate self-care and well-being. Your lower body is the foundation that supports you every step of the way, and these stretches are a beautiful way to honor and nurture it.

In the upcoming chapters, we will explore additional stretches that will enhance your core strength, balance, and overall vitality. Keep embracing this journey with curiosity and self-compassion. Your body will continue to thank you for the love and attention you give it. Let's continue our stretching adventure together!

Core Strengthening Exercises

In this chapter, we will focus on exercises that will fortify your *core muscles*—a crucial foundation for stability, balance, and overall strength. The core encompasses the abdominal muscles and the lower back, working together to support your posture and everyday movements. Let's embark on this empowering journey of core strengthening exercises.

1. Abdominal Strengthening Workouts:

a. **Plank:** Begin in a push-up position with your hands directly beneath your shoulders and your toes on the ground. Engage your core and hold this position for as long as you comfortably can. Keep your body in a straight line from head to heels. Start with shorter holds and gradually increase the duration as you progress.

b. **Bicycle Crunches:** Lie on your back with your hands behind your head and your knees bent. Lift your head, shoulders, and feet off the ground. Bring your right elbow towards your left knee while straightening your right leg. Then switch, bringing your left elbow towards your right knee. Continue alternating in a bicycle pedaling motion.

a. **Superman:** Lie face down on the ground with your arms extended in front of you. Lift your arms, chest, and legs off the ground simultaneously, arching your back slightly. Hold for a few seconds, then lower back down. This exercise strengthens your lower back muscles.

b. **Bridge:** Lie on your back with your knees bent and feet flat on the floor. Place your arms by your sides. Lift your hips off the ground, forming a straight line from your shoulders to your knees. Hold for a moment, then lower back down. This exercise targets your lower back and gluteal muscles.

As you engage in these core strengthening exercises, focus on maintaining proper form and breathing steadily throughout each movement. Avoid straining your neck or lower back and listen to your body's cues. Gradually increase the intensity and duration of the exercises as your core strength improves.

Your core serves as the pillar of support for your body, aiding in daily activities and improving balance. Strengthening these muscles will not only enhance your physical performance but also contribute to a healthier, more stable posture.

Let's continue to explore various stretching and strengthening exercises that will contribute to your overall fitness and well-being. Keep embracing this journey with dedication and self-compassion. Each step you take in this empowering adventure brings you closer to a more vibrant and resilient you. Let's continue our stretching and strengthening journey together!

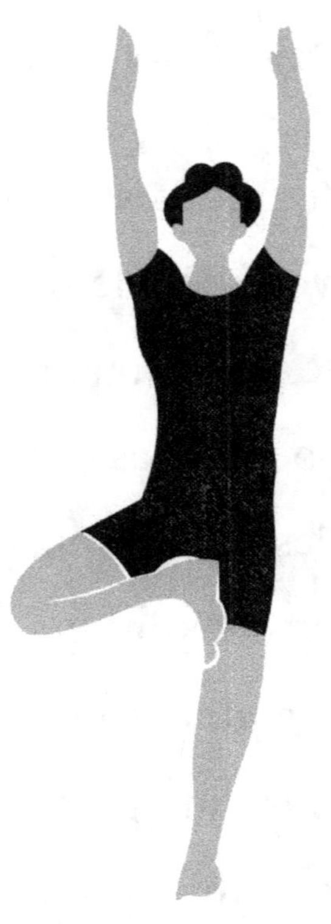

Balance and Flexibility Training

Let's dive into the realms of balance and flexibility—two key elements that play a significant role in maintaining mobility and overall well-being as we age. These exercises are designed to enhance your sense of balance and flexibility, contributing to better stability and a more agile body. Let's embark on this invigorating journey of balance and flexibility training.

1. Balance Exercises for Seniors:

a. **Single Leg Stance:** Stand tall and shift your weight onto one leg while lifting the other slightly off the ground. Find a focal point in front of you to help with balance. Hold this position for as long as you comfortably can, then switch to the other leg. Use a wall or chair for support if needed.

b. **Heel-to-Toe Walk:** Imagine walking on a tightrope. Place the heel of one foot directly in front of the toes of the other foot with each step. This exercise challenges your balance and coordination.

2. Enhancing Flexibility for Daily Activities:

a. **Toe Touches:** Stand with your feet hip-width apart. Slowly bend at the waist, reaching your hands towards your toes or the floor. Let your head hang gently. Hold for a few seconds, feeling the stretch along your hamstrings and lower back.

b. **Seated Forward Fold:** Sit on the edge of a chair with your feet flat on the floor. Gently hinge at your hips and fold forward, reaching towards your feet or ankles. This stretch enhances hamstring and lower back flexibility.

As you engage in these balance and flexibility exercises, focus on maintaining steady breath and being present in each movement. Remember that balance and flexibility are skills that can be developed over time with consistent practice. It's important to prioritize safety, so use support when needed and perform these exercises on a stable surface.

The ability to maintain balance and move with flexibility is a gift that enhances your quality of life. These exercises not only improve physical function but also instill a sense of confidence in navigating daily activities with ease.

Embrace each moment of this journey with dedication and self-compassion. Each practice brings you closer to a more balanced, flexible, and vibrant version of yourself. Let's continue our empowering journey of balance and flexibility training together!

you've GOT this!

Full-Body Stretching Workouts

Now, we'll bring together the elements of stretching we've explored so far to create full-body routines that invigorate your entire being. These complete workouts are designed to enhance your health, flexibility, and vitality by targeting various muscle groups and promoting overall well-being. Let's embark on this comprehensive journey of full-body stretching workouts.

Each routine combines stretches from different parts of the body, providing a balanced approach to enhancing your flexibility and mobility. Follow along with these workouts to enjoy a holistic experience that leaves you feeling refreshed and rejuvenated.

Morning Revival

1. Start with a few minutes of deep, conscious breathing to center yourself.

2. Perform gentle neck rolls and shoulder circles to warm up your upper body.

3. Move on to arm and wrist stretches to release tension in your upper limbs.

4. Gradually transition into hip and thigh stretches to awaken your lower body.

5. Engage in leg and calf stretches to improve lower body flexibility.

6. Conclude with ankle and foot stretches to maintain mobility in your feet.

7. Finish the routine with a few moments of mindful breathing and gratitude.

Evening Relaxation

1. Begin with calming breaths to relax your mind and body.

2. Progress through gentle spinal twists to release tension in your back.

3. Perform chest and shoulder stretches to open up your upper body.

4. Move on to hamstring and lower back stretches to ease any discomfort.

5. Engage in balance exercises to promote stability and focus.

6. Conclude the routine with soothing neck and shoulder stretches.

7. Take a moment to relax in a seated position and appreciate your efforts.

By incorporating these full-body stretching routines into your daily or weekly schedule, you'll experience improved overall health, enhanced flexibility, and a greater sense of vitality. The combination of stretches from head to toe ensures that every muscle group is cared for, leaving you with a feeling of well-being that resonates throughout your day.

Remember that consistency is key. As you practice these routines, you'll likely notice increased mobility, reduced stiffness, and a greater sense of harmony between your body and mind. Enjoy the journey of discovering the transformative effects of full-body stretching workouts.

Let's continue our empowering journey of holistic health and vitality together!

Cool Down and Relaxation

Together, we'll explore the art of cooling down and finding tranquility after your workout. These relaxing stretches and mindful breathing techniques are designed to ease your body and mind, allowing you to embrace a sense of calm and rejuvenation. Let's embark on this soothing journey of cool down and relaxation.

RELAXING STRETCHES TO WIND DOWN AFTER A WORKOUT:

1. **Child's Pose:** Begin on your hands and knees, then sit back on your heels while extending your arms forward. Allow your

forehead to rest on the ground. Feel the gentle stretch in your back and hips.

2. **Seated Forward Fold:** Sit with your legs extended in front of you. Gently hinge at your hips and reach forward, aiming to touch your toes or shins. Let your head hang for a soothing stretch.

3. **Supine Spinal Twist:** Lie on your back, hug your knees to your chest, then let them fall to one side. Extend your arms out in a T shape and gaze in the opposite direction. This twist releases tension in your spine.

1. **Box Breathing:** Inhale for a count of 4, hold for a count of 4, exhale for a count of 4, and hold for a count of 4. Repeat this pattern several times. Focus on the rhythm of your breath and let go of any tension.

2. **Belly Breathing:** Place one hand on your chest and the other on your belly. Inhale deeply through your nose, allowing your belly to rise. Exhale slowly through your mouth, feeling your belly fall. This technique promotes relaxation.

3. **Guided Visualization:** Close your eyes and imagine a peaceful place—a beach, a

forest, or a calming meadow. Breathe deeply as you visualize yourself in this serene environment, letting go of stress with each breath.

As you engage in these cool-down stretches and breathing techniques, allow yourself to fully unwind. The transition from active movement to stillness is a sacred moment to honor your body's efforts and embrace a state of tranquility. These practices not only enhance your physical recovery but also nurture your mental and emotional well-being.

Keep embracing this journey with patience and self compassion. Every step you take towards relaxation and self-care brings you closer to a more peaceful and vibrant version of yourself. Let's continue our journey of cool down and relaxation together!

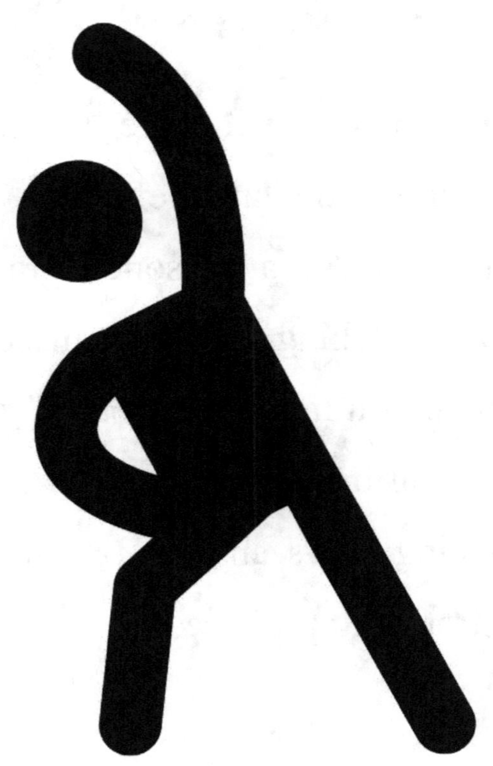

Tips for Safe Stretching

In this chapter, we'll delve into essential tips to ensure safe and effective stretching. Whether you're a seasoned practitioner or new to stretching exercises, these guidelines will help you make the most of your routine while prioritizing your safety and well-being. Let's embark on this journey of safe stretching practices.

Common Mistakes to Avoid:

1. **Overstretching:** Avoid pushing your body beyond its comfortable range of motion. Stretching should feel like a gentle pull, not pain.

2. **Bouncing**: Never bounce during a stretch. Instead, perform smooth and controlled movements to prevent injury.

3. **Holding Your Breath:**
Maintain steady breathing throughout each stretch. Deep breaths help relax your muscles and enhance the stretch's effectiveness.

4. **Neglecting Warm-Up:** Always warm up your body before stretching. Cold muscles are more prone to injury.

5. **Ignoring Pain:** Discomfort is normal, but if you feel pain during a stretch, stop immediately and reassess your form.

1. **Consult Your Doctor:** If you have any medical conditions or concerns, consult your healthcare provider before starting a new stretching routine.

2. **Start Slowly:** Begin with gentle stretches and gradually increase intensity. Listen to your body and progress at a pace that feels comfortable.

3. **Use Support:** If needed, use a chair, wall, or other stable surface for support during balance exercises or deeper stretches.

4. **Stay Hydrated:** Drink water before and after your routine to stay hydrated, aiding muscle function and overall well-being.

5. **Maintain Balance:** Focus on balance exercises that challenge you without compromising your safety. Use a chair or rail for support if necessary.

6. **Adapt Stretches:** Modify stretches to suit your body's needs and limitations. There's no need to force a particular pose if it doesn't feel right.

As you engage in your stretching routine, remember that your safety and comfort are paramount. Stretching should be an enjoyable experience that nurtures your body and promotes overall well-being. By following these tips and safety considerations, you'll create a foundation of self-care that will serve you well on your journey to improved health and flexibility.

With each stretch, you're investing in a healthier and more vibrant you. Let's continue our journey of safe and effective stretching together!

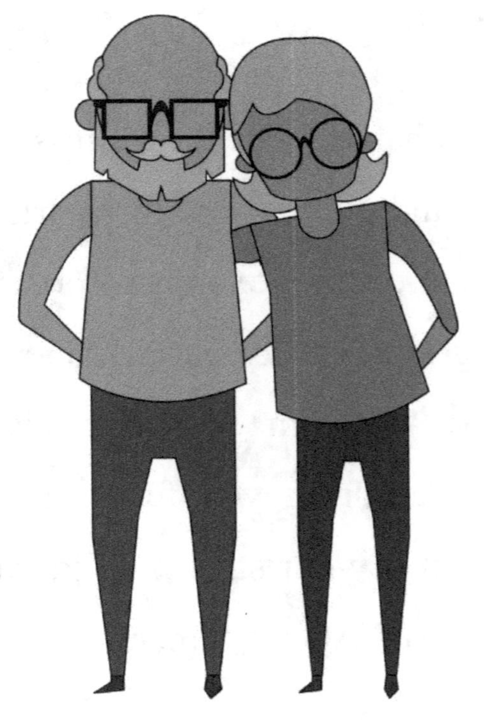

Frequently Asked Questions (FAQs)

In this chapter, we'll address common concerns and queries that often arise when it comes to stretching exercises for seniors. By providing answers to these frequently asked questions, we aim to offer clarity and guidance, ensuring you feel confident and empowered in your stretching journey. Let's explore these FAQs together.

Q1: How often should I stretch?

A: Ideally, aim for at least 3 to 5 days of stretching per week. Consistency is key for improved flexibility and overall well-being.

However, always listen to your body and give yourself rest days if needed.

Q2: Can I stretch if I have joint pain or arthritis?

A: Yes, but with caution. Gentle stretching can help alleviate joint discomfort. Focus on low-impact stretches and consult your healthcare provider before starting a new routine.

Q3: What's the best time to stretch?

A: You can stretch at any time of the day that suits you. Some prefer morning stretches to awaken the body, while others find evening stretches help them unwind before bed.

Q4: How long should I hold a stretch?

A: Aim to hold each stretch for 15 to 30 seconds. This allows your muscles to relax and lengthen gradually.

Q5: Can I stretch after a workout?

A: Yes, post-workout stretching can help relax your muscles and prevent stiffness. Focus on static stretches during this time.

Q6: Should I feel pain during a stretch?

A: No, you should never feel pain. A gentle pull or mild discomfort is normal, but if you experience pain, ease out of the stretch immediately.

Q7: Can stretching help with balance and stability?

A: Absolutely. Many stretching exercises also improve balance by engaging core muscles and enhancing body awareness.

Q8: Can I modify stretches if they're too difficult?

A: Yes, absolutely. Modify stretches to match your current flexibility and comfort level. Use props or support as needed.

Q9: Is there an age limit for stretching exercises?

A: There's no age limit. Stretching is beneficial for people of all ages. Just ensure you choose stretches that suit your body's needs and limitations.

Q10: Can I do more advanced stretches over time?

A: Yes, as your flexibility improves, you can gradually introduce more advanced stretches. Always prioritize safety and proper form.

Remember, these answers are meant to guide you, but each person's body is unique. If you have specific concerns or questions, consider consulting a healthcare provider or fitness professional. The journey of stretching exercises is about discovering what works best for you and nurturing your body's well-being.

Conclusion

As we conclude our journey through ***"Stretching Exercises for Seniors,"*** let's reflect on the remarkable benefits that stretching offers to enhance your health, vitality, and overall well-being. Throughout this book, we've explored various stretches, exercises, and mindfulness techniques, all designed to empower you on your path to a healthier and more fulfilling life.

Summary of the Benefits of Stretching Exercises for Seniors:

1. **Improved Flexibility:** Regular stretching increases your range of motion, making

everyday movements easier and more comfortable.

2. **Enhanced Mobility:** By keeping your muscles and joints supple, stretching helps maintain your ability to perform daily tasks with ease.

3. **Better Posture:** Stretching exercises strengthen your core muscles and encourage proper alignment, leading to improved posture and reduced strain on your body.

4. **Pain Relief:** Stretching can alleviate muscle tension and discomfort, offering relief from nagging aches and pains associated with aging.

5. **Stress Reduction:** Mindful breathing and relaxation techniques incorporated into stretching routines promote mental clarity and emotional well-being.

6. **Balanced Body:** Incorporating balance exercises in your routine enhances stability, reducing the risk of falls and injuries.

7. **Core Strength:** Strengthening your core muscles through targeted exercises supports your spine and promotes overall strength.

8. **Quality of Life:** As you experience improved mobility, reduced discomfort, and

enhanced vitality, your overall quality of life improves.

As you embrace the benefits of stretching exercises, remember that this journey is about more than just physical movement. It's a journey of self-discovery, self-care, and empowerment. Each stretch is an act of love towards your body—a way of honoring the wisdom it holds and the journey it has taken.

While the final chapter of this book marks the end of its pages, it marks only the beginning of your stretching adventure. Carry the lessons, exercises, and mindfulness practices with you as you continue on your path to a healthier, more vibrant life. Embrace each day as an opportunity to stretch not only your body but also your limits, reaching for new levels of well-being and vitality.

Thank you for joining us on this empowering journey through ***"Stretching Exercises for Seniors."*** May you continue to find guidance, joy, strength, and inspiration in every stretch you undertake. Let the wisdom of stretching guide you towards a life filled with balance, flexibility, and boundless possibilities.

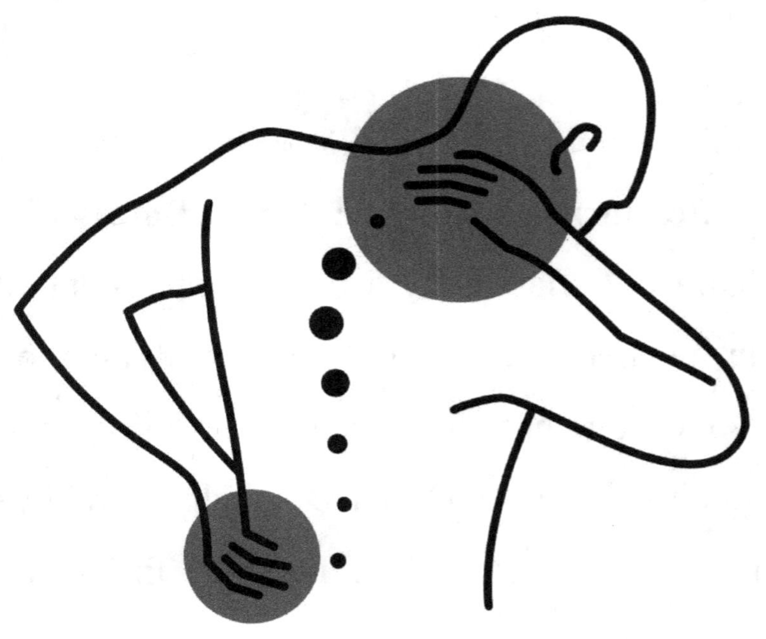

Bonus: 20 Free Pain Relief Balm Recipes

1. **Peppermint and Eucalyptus Balm:** This balm is a classic for a reason. The menthol in peppermint oil and the eucalyptus oil work together to create a cooling and soothing sensation that can help to relieve pain and inflammation. To make this balm, you will need:

* 1 cup of coconut oil, melted

* 1/4 cup of beeswax, melted

* 10 drops of peppermint essential oil

* 10 drops of eucalyptus essential oil

* 10 drops of lavender essential oil (optional)

Instructions:

1. Combine the coconut oil and beeswax in a double boiler over low heat.

2. Once the beeswax is melted, remove the mixture from the heat and stir in the essential oils.

3. Pour the mixture into a glass jar and let it cool completely.

2. **Arnica Balm:** Arnica is a well-known herb for pain relief. It is often used to treat bruises, sprains, and muscle pain. To make an arnica balm, you will need:

   * 1 cup of shea butter, melted
   * 1/4 cup of coconut oil, melted
   * 1 tablespoon of arnica tincture
   * 10 drops of lavender essential oil

Instructions:

1. Combine the shea butter, coconut oil, and arnica tincture in a double boiler over low heat.

2. Once the mixture is melted, remove it from the heat and stir in the lavender essential oil.

3. Pour the mixture into a glass jar and let it cool completely.

3. **Camphor Balm:** Camphor is a topical analgesic that can help to relieve pain and inflammation. It is often used to treat muscle pain, arthritis, and headaches. To make a camphor balm, you will need:

* 1 cup of coconut oil, melted
* 1/4 cup of beeswax, melted

* 1 tablespoon of camphor oil

* 10 drops of peppermint essential oil

Instructions:

1. Combine the coconut oil, beeswax, and camphor oil in a double boiler over low heat.

2. Once the mixture is melted, remove it from the heat and stir in the peppermint essential oil.

3. Pour the mixture into a glass jar and let it cool completely.

4. **Wheatgrass Balm:** Wheatgrass is a good source of vitamins and minerals, including vitamins A, C, E, and K. It also contains antioxidants that can help to reduce

inflammation. To make a wheatgrass balm, you will need:

    * 1 cup of wheatgrass juice

    * 1/4 cup of coconut oil, melted

    * 1/4 cup of beeswax, melted

    * 10 drops of lavender essential oil

Instructions:

1. Combine the wheatgrass juice, coconut oil, and beeswax in a double boiler over low heat.

2. Once the mixture is melted, remove it from the heat and stir in the lavender essential oil.

3. Pour the mixture into a glass jar and let it cool completely.

5. **Clove Balm:** Clove oil is a natural pain reliever that can help to relieve toothache pain, muscle pain, and arthritis pain. To make a clove balm, you will need:

    * 1 cup of coconut oil, melted

    * 1/4 cup of beeswax, melted

    * 10 drops of clove essential oil

    * 10 drops of peppermint essential oil

Instructions:

1. Combine the coconut oil, beeswax, and clove essential oil in a double boiler over low heat.

2. Once the mixture is melted, remove it from the heat and stir in the peppermint essential oil.

3. Pour the mixture into a glass jar and let it cool completely.

6. **Turmeric Balm:** Turmeric is a spice that has anti-inflammatory and pain-relieving properties. It is often used to treat arthritis, muscle pain, and joint pain. To make a turmeric balm, you will need:

    * 1 cup of coconut oil, melted

    * 1/4 cup of beeswax, melted

    * 1 tablespoon of turmeric powder

    * 10 drops of ginger essential oil

Instructions:

1. Combine the coconut oil, beeswax, and turmeric powder in a double boiler over low heat.

2. Once the mixture is melted, remove it from the heat and stir in the ginger essential oil.

3. Pour the mixture into a glass jar and let it cool

7. **Lavender Balm:** Lavender is a calming and relaxing essential oil that can also help to relieve pain. It is often used to treat headaches, muscle pain, and anxiety. To make a lavender balm, you will need:

* 1 cup of coconut oil, melted
* 1/4 cup of beeswax, melted
* 10 drops of lavender essential oil

8. **Rosemary balm:**

Ingredients:

* 1 cup of coconut oil, melted

* 1/4 cup of beeswax, melted

* 10 drops of rosemary essential oil

Instructions:

1. Combine the coconut oil and beeswax in a double boiler over low heat.

2. Once the beeswax is melted, remove the mixture from the heat and stir in the rosemary essential oil.

3. Pour the mixture into a glass jar and let it cool completely.

9. **Eucalyptus Balm:** Eucalyptus is a refreshing and decongestant essential oil that can help to relieve pain and open up the airways. It is often used to treat sinus pain,

headaches, and muscle pain. To make an eucalyptus balm, you will need:

    * 1 cup of coconut oil, melted

    * 1/4 cup of beeswax, melted

    * 10 drops of eucalyptus essential oil

10. **Wintergreen Balm:** Wintergreen is a topical analgesic that can help to relieve pain and inflammation. It is often used to treat muscle pain, arthritis, and headaches. To make a wintergreen balm, you will need:

    * 1 cup of coconut oil, melted

    * 1/4 cup of beeswax, melted

    * 1 tablespoon of wintergreen oil

11. **Tea Tree Balm:** Tea tree oil is an antiseptic and antibacterial essential oil that

can help to relieve pain and infection. It is often used to treat cuts, bruises, and acne. To make a tea tree balm, you will need:

* 1 cup of coconut oil, melted
* 1/4 cup of beeswax, melted
* 10 drops of tea tree essential oil

12. **Frankincense Balm:** Frankincense is a calming and relaxing essential oil that can also help to relieve pain. It is often used to treat headaches, muscle pain, and anxiety. To make a frankincense balm, you will need:

* 1 cup of coconut oil, melted
* 1/4 cup of beeswax, melted
* 10 drops of frankincense essential oil

13. **Myrrh Balm:** Myrrh is a pain-relieving and anti-inflammatory essential oil that can help to relieve pain and inflammation. It is often used to treat arthritis, muscle pain, and joint pain. To make a myrrh balm, you will need:

* 1 cup of coconut oil, melted
* 1/4 cup of beeswax, melted
* 10 drops of myrrh essential oil

14. **Chamomile Balm:** Chamomile is a calming and relaxing essential oil that can also help to relieve pain. It is often used to treat headaches, muscle pain, and anxiety. To make a chamomile balm, you will need:

* 1 cup of coconut oil, melted
* 1/4 cup of beeswax, melted

* 10 drops of chamomile essential oil

15. **Oregano Balm:** Oregano is an antiseptic and antibacterial essential oil that can help to relieve pain and infection. It is often used to treat cuts, bruises, and acne. To make an oregano balm, you will need:
    * 1 cup of coconut oil, melted
    * 1/4 cup of beeswax, melted
    * 10 drops of oregano essential oil

16. **Peppermint and Ginger Balm:** This balm combines the cooling and soothing effects of peppermint oil with the warming and invigorating effects of ginger oil. It is a great balm for relieving muscle pain,

arthritis pain, and headaches. To make this balm, you will need:

 * 1 cup of coconut oil, melted

 * 1/4 cup of beeswax, melted

 * 10 drops of peppermint essential oil

 * 10 drops of ginger essential oil

17. **Lavender and Chamomile Balm:** This balm combines the calming and relaxing effects of lavender oil with the soothing effects of chamomile oil. It is a great balm for relieving stress, anxiety, and insomnia.

Ingredients:

* 1 cup of coconut oil, melted

* 1/4 cup of beeswax, melted

* 10 drops of lavender essential oil

* 10 drops of chamomile essential oil

Instructions:

1. Combine the coconut oil and beeswax in a double boiler over low heat.

2. Once the beeswax is melted, remove the mixture from the heat and stir in the lavender and chamomile essential oils.

3. Pour the mixture into a glass jar and let it cool completely.

18. **Eucalyptus and Rosemary Balm:** This balm combines the refreshing and decongestant effects of eucalyptus oil with the stimulating effects of rosemary oil. It is a great balm for relieving sinus pain, headaches, and muscle pain. To make this balm, you will need:

* 1 cup of coconut oil, melted

* 1/4 cup of beeswax, melted

* 10 drops of eucalyptus essential oil

* 10 drops of rosemary essential oil

19. **Wintergreen and Tea Tree Balm:** This balm combines the topical analgesic effects of wintergreen oil with the antiseptic and antibacterial effects of tea tree oil. It is a great balm for relieving muscle pain, arthritis pain, and headaches. To make this balm, you will need:

* 1 cup of coconut oil, melted

* 1/4 cup of beeswax, melted

* 1 tablespoon of wintergreen oil

* 10 drops of tea tree essential oil

20. **Frankincense, Myrrh, and Chamomile Balm:** This balm combines the calming and relaxing effects of frankincense and chamomile oils with the pain-relieving and anti-inflammatory effects of myrrh oil. It is a great balm for relieving pain and inflammation, as well as stress and anxiety. To make this balm, you will need:

   * 1 cup of coconut oil, melted
   * 1/4 cup of beeswax, melted
   * 10 drops of frankincense essential oil
   * 10 drops of myrrh essential oil
   * 10 drops of chamomile essential oil

* Use high-quality ingredients, such as organic coconut oil and beeswax.

* Use essential oils that are appropriate for the type of pain you are trying to relieve.

* Start with a small amount of essential oil and increase the amount as needed.

* Test the balm on a small area of skin before applying it to a large area.

* Store the balm in a cool, dark place.

Pain relief balms can be a great way to relieve pain and inflammation naturally. They are easy to make and use, and they can be customized to your specific needs.

www.ingramcontent.com/pod-product-compliance
Lightning Source LLC
Chambersburg PA
CBHW070840260726
48660CB00005B/2096